While planning to achieve fitness goals, it is almost certain that starting and sticking to a healthy plan can sometimes seem impossible.

Often, people simply tend to face two things which are the motivation to get started or lose their motivation to keep going. Luckily, motivation is something you can work to increase.

I have carefully written 30 ways that can make you smash your fitness challenge and motivate yourself to finish strong.

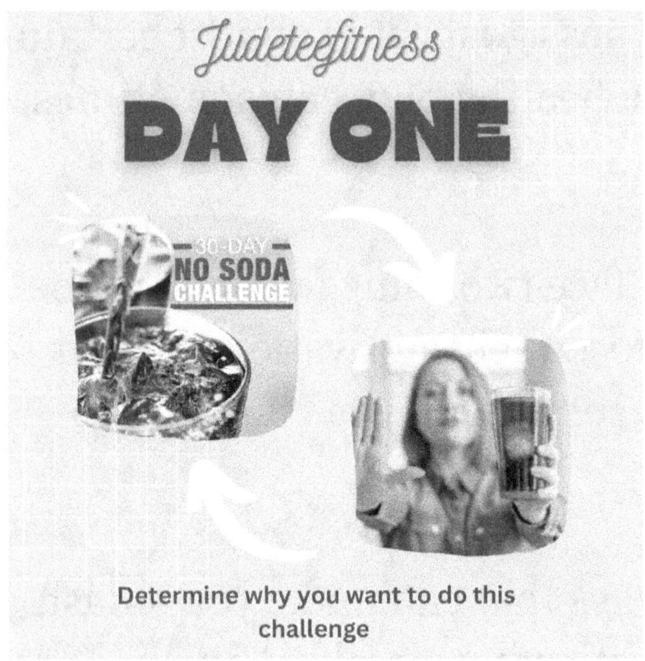

DAY ONE

Determine Why You Want to Do This Challenge

Clearly define all the reasons you want to do the no soda challenge and write them down. This will help you stay committed and motivated to reach your goals.

Try to read through them daily and use them as a reminder when tempted to drink soda.

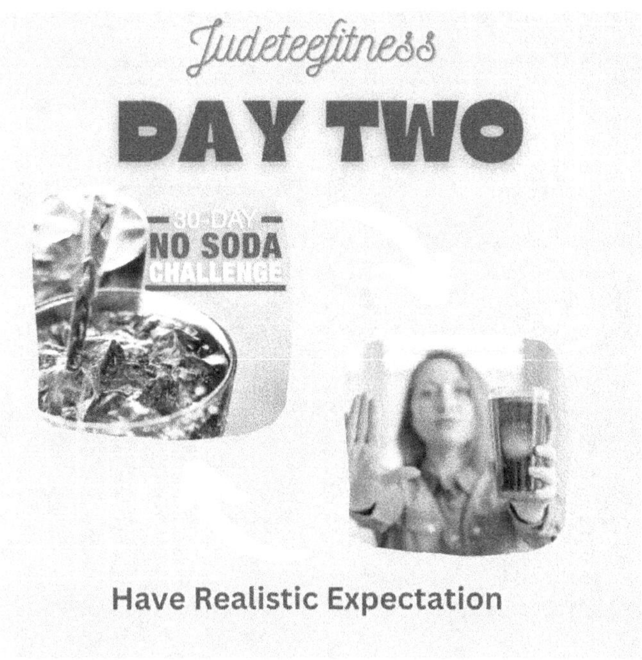

DAY TWO

Have Realistic Expectations

Trust me, setting unattainable goals can lead to feelings of frustration and cause you to give up. On the contrary, setting and accomplishing achievable goals leads to feelings of accomplishment.

People who reach their self determined goals are more likely to maintain their fitness long-term goals.

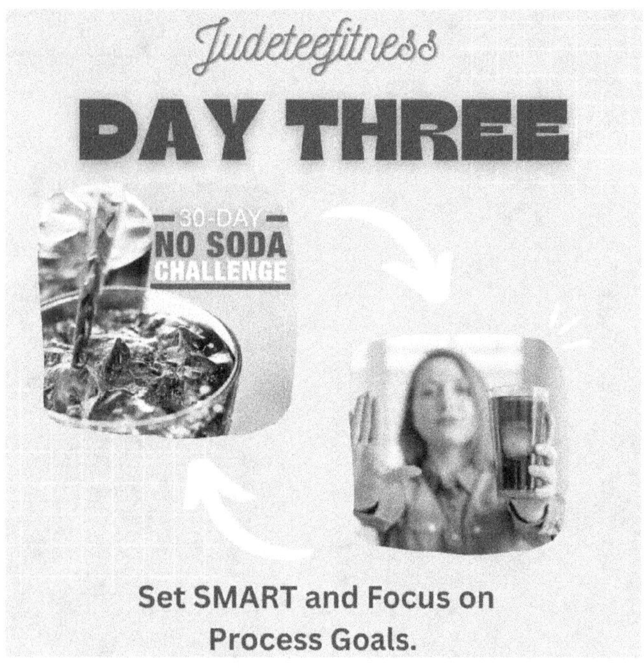

DAY THREE.

Set SMART and Focus on Process Goals.

Many people trying to do any form of fitness challenge like the one we are currently doing only set outcome goals or goals they want to accomplish at the end of a certain period. Unfortunately, do you know that focusing only on outcome goals can derail your motivation? This is because they may feel too distant and leave you feeling overwhelmed.

Instead, I encourage you to set SMART process goals or activities you are going to take to reach your desired/final goals. A perfect example of a process goal is exercising at least three times a week.

NOTE: setting SMART process goals will help you stay motivated while focusing only on outcome goals can lead to disappointment and lessen your motivation.

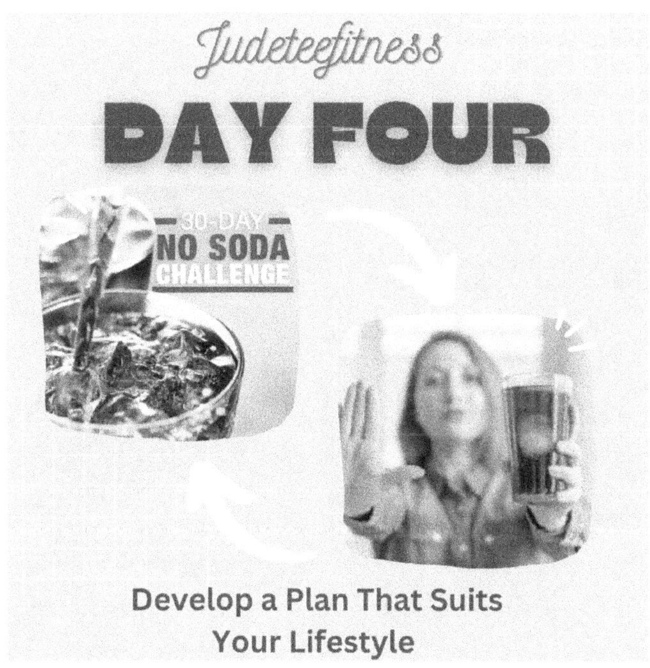

DAY FOUR

Develop a Plan That Suits Your Lifestyle

During this period your body will crave soda especially when you are with people who take it or see it often. Find a plan that you can stick to, and avoid plans that would be nearly impossible to follow in the long term.

Consider creating a custom plan that best suits your lifestyle. It can be avoiding places where you can easily purchase soda, going for a walk, or getting an accountability partner. Just anything that works for you.

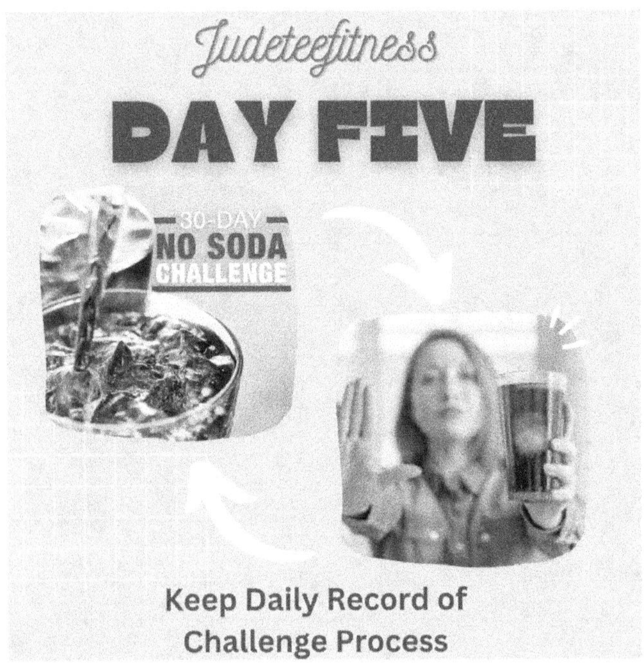

DAY FIVE

Keep Daily Record of Challenge Process

Keeping a record of your daily process, hiccups and hurdles can help you measure progress. Recall that on day two I asked you to share the temptations you encountered. Some did and some did not. However, It is important to identify triggers and hold yourself accountable.

Self-monitoring is crucial to overcoming this challenge as well as motivation and success. Research has found that people who track their daily processes are more likely to smash their fitness goals.

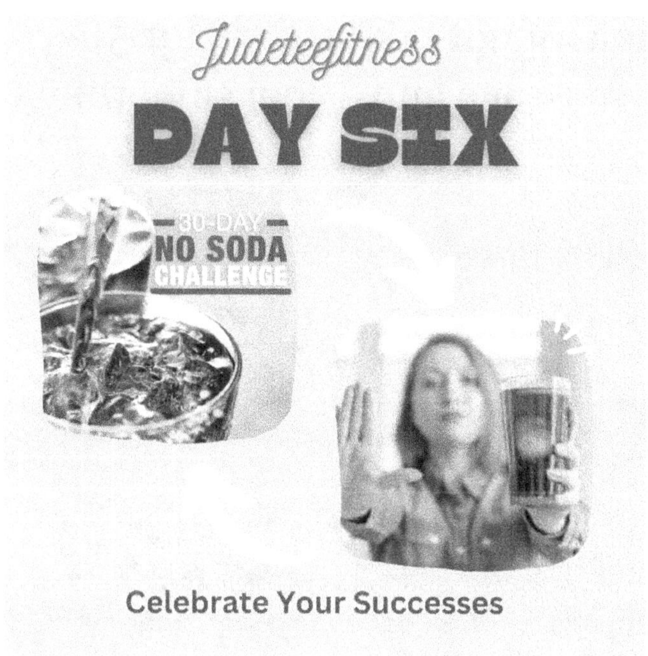

DAY SIX

Celebrate Your Successes

If you are addicted or crave a lot of soda then doing this challenge is hard. So, celebrate all your successes for each day to keep yourself motivated. This applies to our everyday life when we hit a milestone.

Give yourself some credit when you accomplish a goal. In this group, I always encourage you to share your wins over every temptation. When you feel pride in yourself, you will increase your motivation.

Moreover, remember to celebrate behavior changes and not just reach a certain number on the scale.

For example, if you met your goal of not taking soda for 5 days, treat yourself with a nice massage and a cool smoothie or anything fun for you.

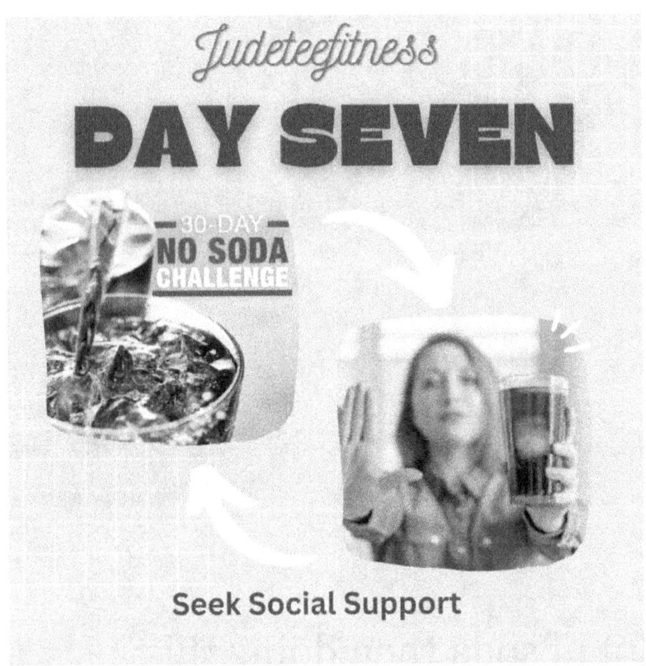

DAY SEVEN

Seek Social Support

Do you know that having strong social support will help hold you accountable and keep you motivated to complete the 30 days no soda challenge? Consider joining a support group to help boost your motivation along the way.

People need regular support and positive feedback to stay motivated. During the 30-day challenge, I took out time to reach out to everyone in the group just to support their goals and commitment.

You can also tell your close family and friends about your goals so they can help support you on your journey. Additionally, it can be helpful to involve your friend or partner who desires to be fit but make sure to get support from other people too, such as your friends(fitness group).

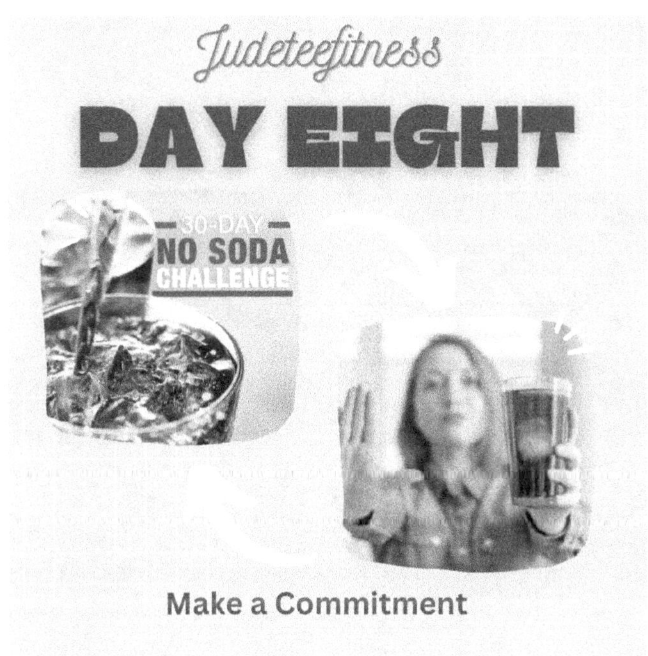

DAY EIGHT

Make a Commitment

Making a public commitment to your fitness goals (challenge) will help you stay motivated and hold you accountable especially to your family and colleagues.

Research shows that those who make a public commitment are more likely to follow through with their goals.
Telling others will help you stay accountable, They act as your accountability partner unknowingly.

Tell your close family and friends, and even consider sharing them on social media. The more people you share your goals with, the greater the accountability.

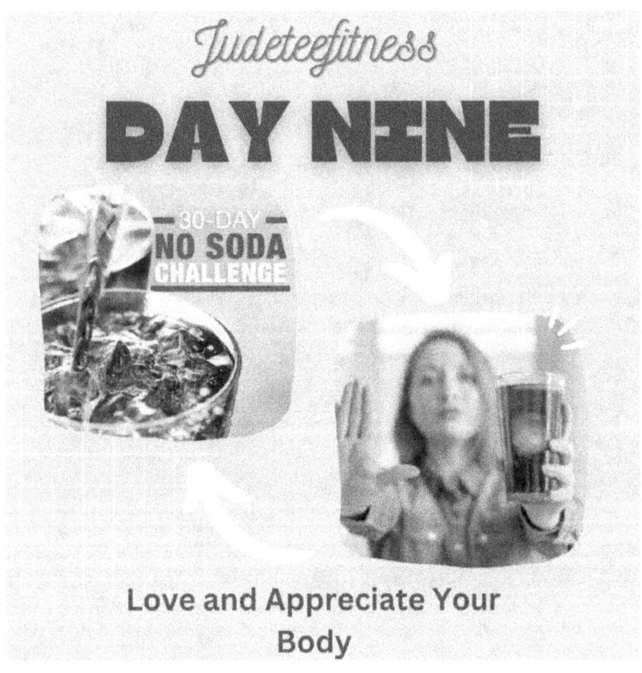

DAY NINE

Love and Appreciate Your Body

One step to achieving great fit is love and appreciation. Research has repeatedly found that people who dislike their bodies are less likely to engage in fitness challenges or lose weight.

However, taking steps to improve yourself can help you smash those challenges and finish one day at a time.
Finally, the following activities can help boost your body image. They include;

1. Exercise
2. Surround yourself with positive people.
3. Avoid comparing yourself to others, especially models.
4. Do something for yourself, such as getting a massage.
5. Wear clothes you like and that fit you well.
6. Look in the mirror and say the things you like about yourself out loud.
7. Appreciate what your body can do.

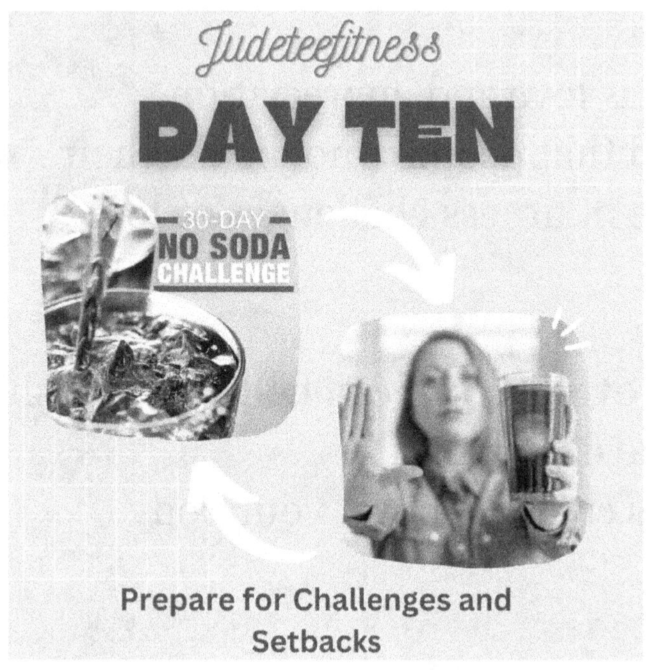

DAY TEN

Prepare for Challenges and Setbacks

As previously stated we have more fitness challenges coming up so get ready for more challenges. However, it is important to know that everyday stressors will always pop up.

Finding ways to plan for them and developing proper coping skills will help you stay motivated no matter what life throws your way. Unfortunately, there will always be holidays, birthdays, or parties that will make soda look you in the eyes. And there will always be stressors at work or with family.

So, It's important to start problem-solving and brainstorming about these possible challenges and setbacks. This will keep you from getting off track and losing motivation

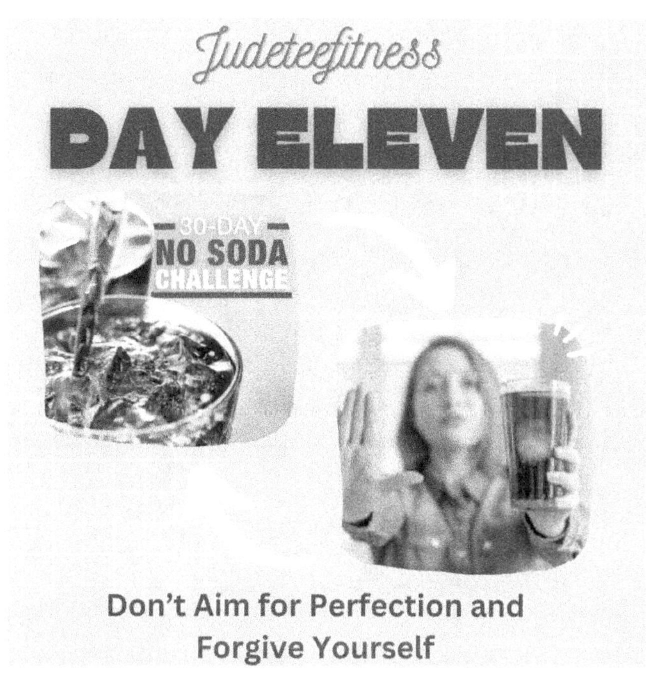

DAY ELEVEN

Don't Aim for Perfection and Forgive Yourself

In my opinion, when you aim for perfection, you will quickly lose your motivation. You do not have to be perfect to smash those goals.

If you have an "all or nothing" approach, you're less likely to achieve your goals.

When you are too restrictive, you may find yourself saying "I have been drinking cold orange and pineapple chivita, so I might as well have a cold Pepsi."

Avoid beating yourself up when you make a mistake. Self-defeating thoughts will just hinder your motivation.

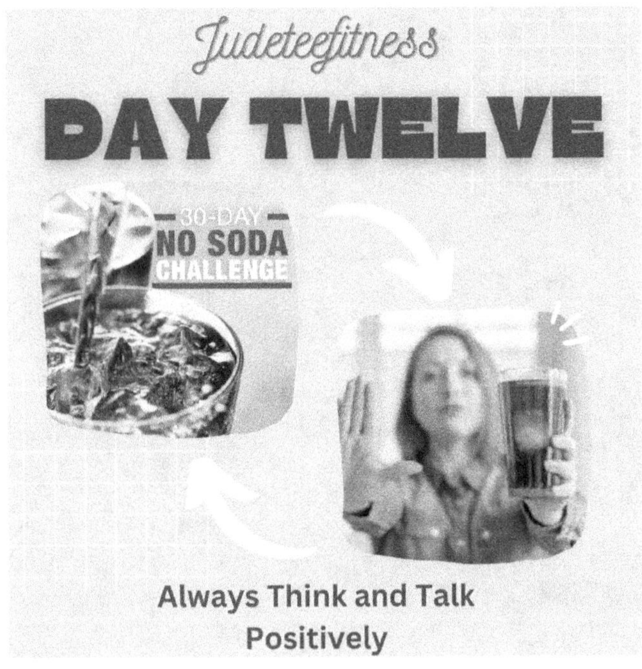

DAY TWELVE

Always Think and Talk Positively

Think and talk positively about your goals, but make sure you are realistic and focus on the steps you must take to reach them. People who have positive expectations and feel confident in their ability to achieve their goals tend to complete the challenge.

Start talking positively about every given challenge. Also, talk about the steps you are going to take and commit your thoughts out loud.

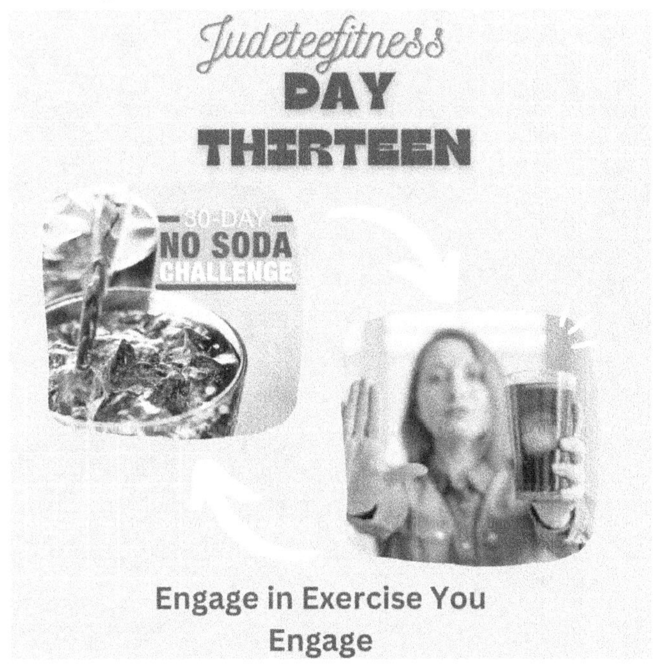

DAY THIRTEEN

Engage In Exercise You Enjoy

The truth remains that exercise not only helps you burn calorics but also makcs you fccl bcttcr. Find an cxcrcisc you enjoy, so it can easily become part of your routine.
Physical activity is an important part of any fitness challenge. Not only does it help you burn calories, but it also improves your well-being and mental state.

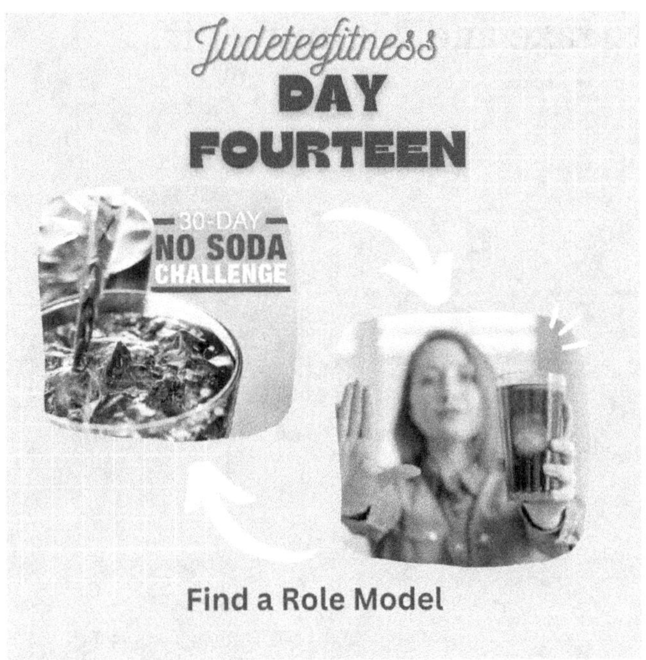

DAY FOURTEEN

Find a Role Model

When trying to accomplish a given task or challenge, you can find a role model. Finding a role model will help keep you motivated. Someone you can relate to. According to the National Institute of Health, having a relatable and positive role model may help keep you motivated.

Maybe you know a friend who has done this before or who is good at it and can be your inspiration. You can also look for inspirational blogs or stories about people who have completed those challenges.

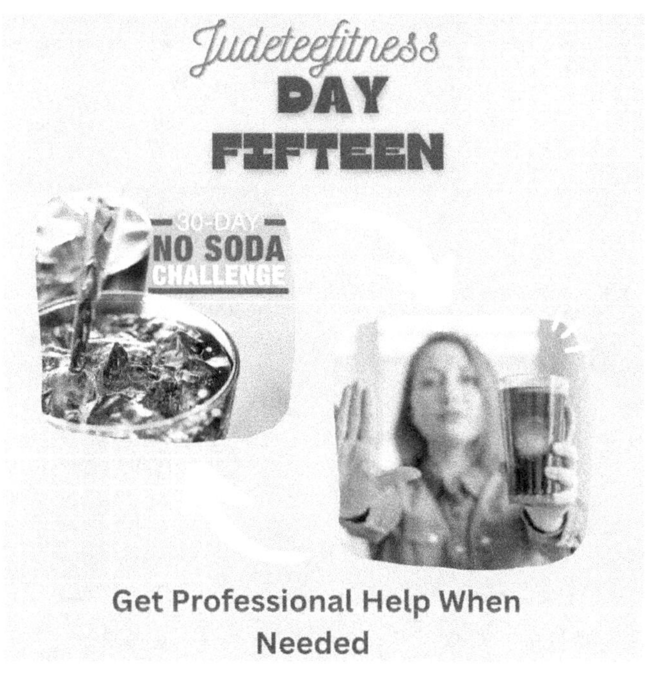

DAY FIFTEEN

Get Professional Help When Needed

Do not hesitate to consult professional help, an expert, or your coach to aid your challenge efforts when needed. People who feel more confident in their knowledge and abilities will lose and smash their goals.

After getting daily tips on how to avoid soda. Let's check out why you should avoid drinking soda.

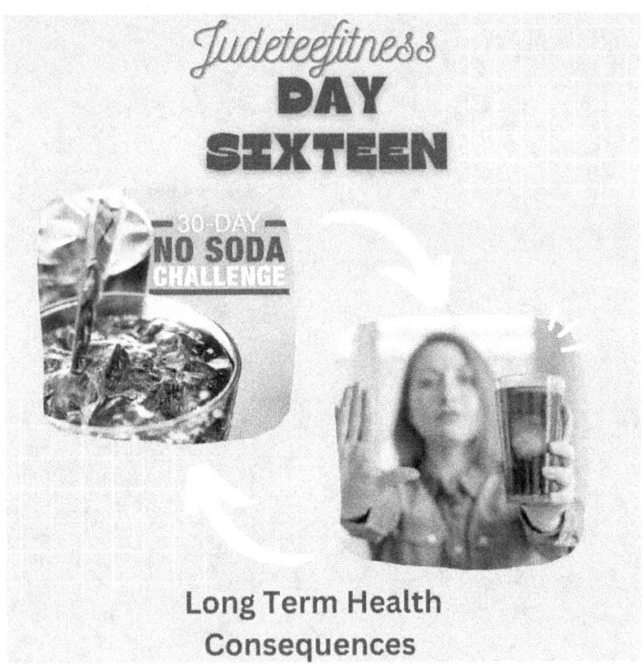

DAY SIXTEEN

Long-term health consequences.

I've listed numerous health reasons to not reduce your intake of soda. So, if you have even one of these health problems because of (or it's exacerbated by) drinking soda, your long-term medical costs will skyrocket. Some of the health reasons include;
1. increases your blood pressure
2. makes you fat
3. destroys your teeth
4. heart disease and diabetes.
5. soda consumption is linked to osteoporosis.

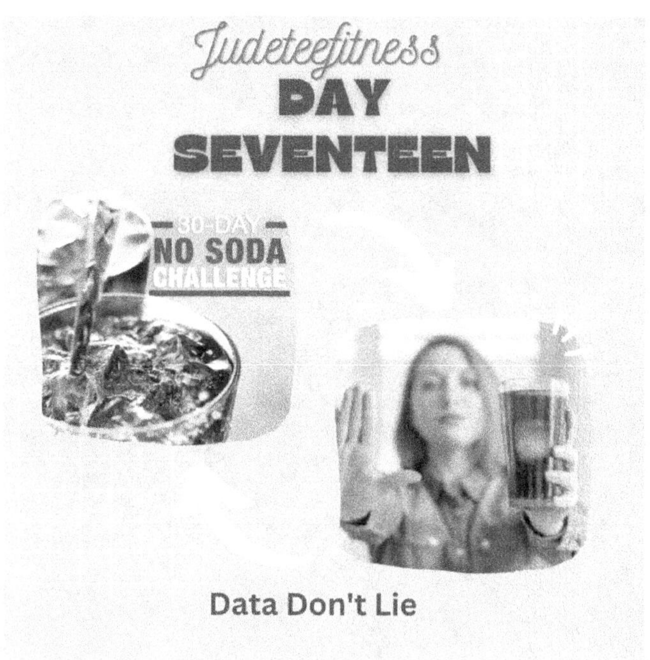

Data Don't Lie

DAY SEVENTEEN

Data Don't Lie.

Trust there are countless studies published with alarming statistics. One study monitored the health of 90,000 women over two decades and found that women who drank two sodas per day had a 40% higher risk of heart disease

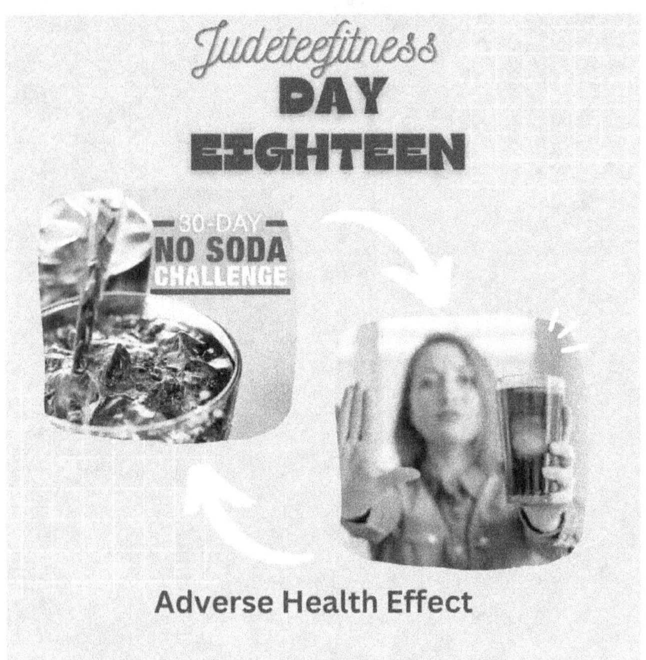

DAY EIGHTEEN

Adverse Health Effect

I recently researched the ingredient lists of some soft drinks and recognized many of the same ingredients that chemical engineers used in the plastics and adhesive industries, some of the chemicals in Coca-Cola are known to increase asthma attacks, skyrocket your glycemic index (chemical sweeteners are 200 times sweeter than table sugar), and cause severe adverse health effects.

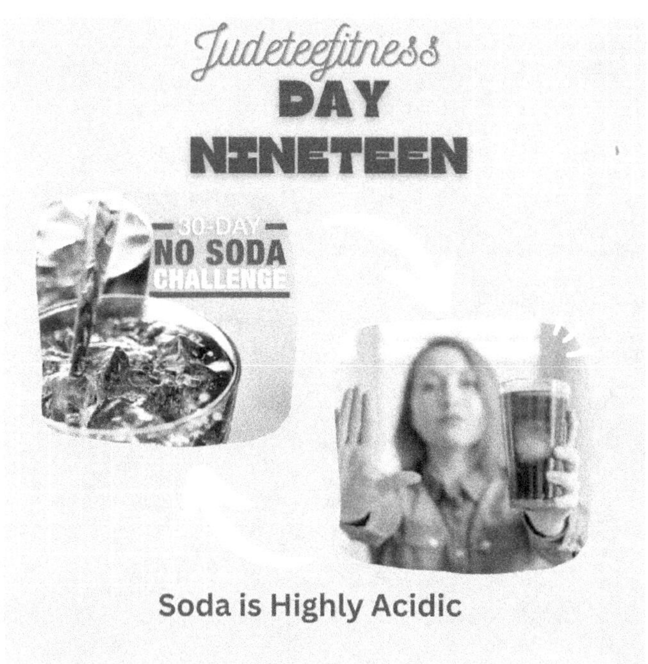

Soda is Highly Acidic

DAY NINETEEN

Soda is Highly Acidic.

Coke is incredibly acidic at a 2.5. The pH of water is a neutral 7. Since the pH scale is logarithmic, that means Coke is 50,000 times more acidic than water.

Also, phosphoric acid interferes with the body's ability to absorb calcium which is critical for bone health.

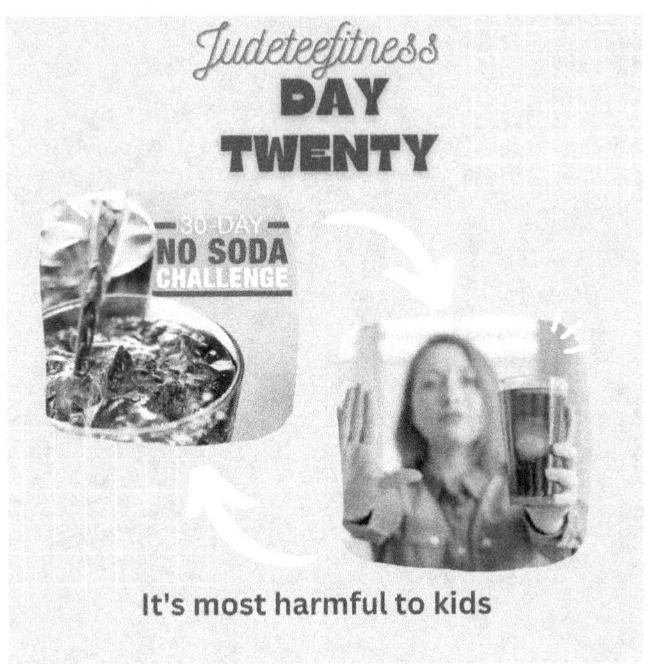

DAY TWENTY

It's Most Harmful to Kids

Try doing your research, you will discover that kids are most targeted by soft drink companies. There are numerous drinks out there that they tag basically for kids. So why try to stay away from soda, you can help a kid too.

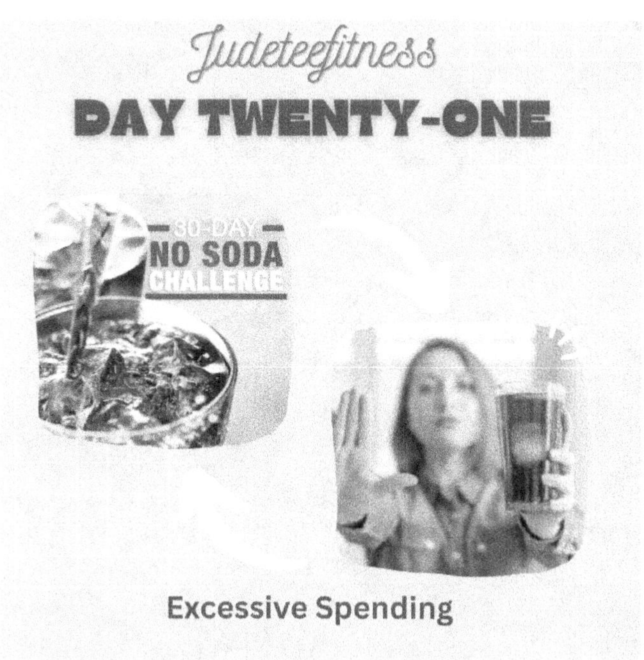

DAY TWENTY-ONE

Excessive Spending

Recently, when I started this challenge I noticed that we waste a lot on what could cause harm to our bodies. That's enough to motivate you to stop or reduce your excessive intake of soda. Studies show that while most Americans know that drinking soda is harmful, 48% of Americans continue to drink an average of 2.6 glasses daily.

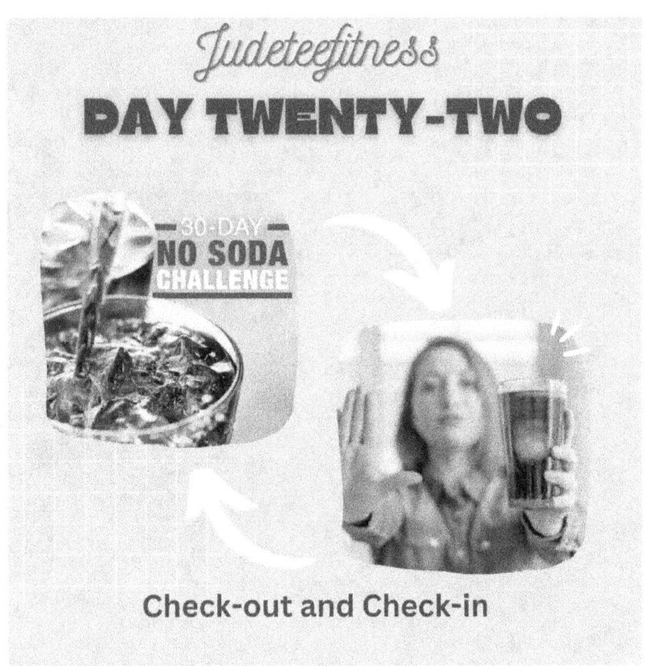

TWENTY-TWO

Check-out and Check-in

I had to say this once again as a little reminder. Avoiding or challenging yourself to certain things, especially one that will help your health comes with a price to pay.
Clean out your fridge and stock it with sparkling water and unsweetened iced tea instead. If you're craving a soda and one is staring you in the face(temptation), you're much more likely to slip.

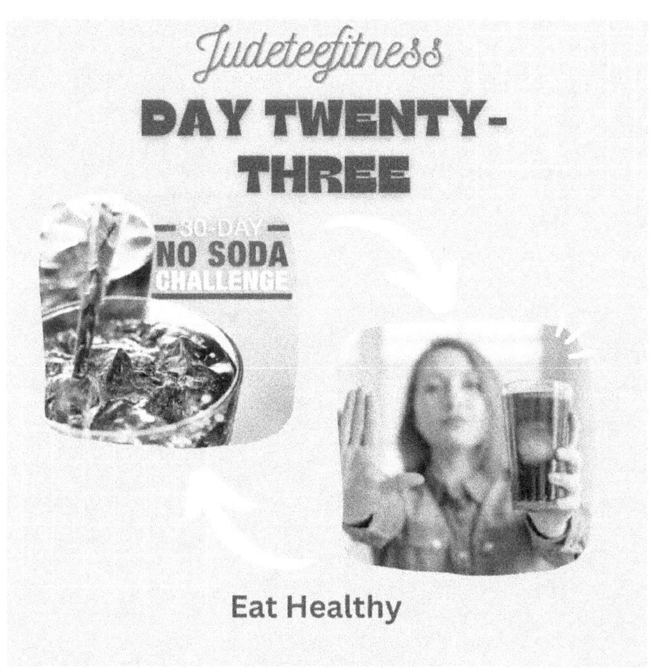

TWENTY-THREE

Eat Healthy

Trust me, this is one part we miss as individuals. However, striving to eat healthy should be encouraged. You can't say you don't want to drink soda but find yourself taking all forms of food.

Eat protein and healthy fats which hclp kccp you full and regulate blood sugar levels; beans, nuts, organic soy products, eggs, yogurt, cheese, fish and avocado are all great sources. Eat solid, nutritious meals to help regulate blood sugar levels, and keep cravings at bay.

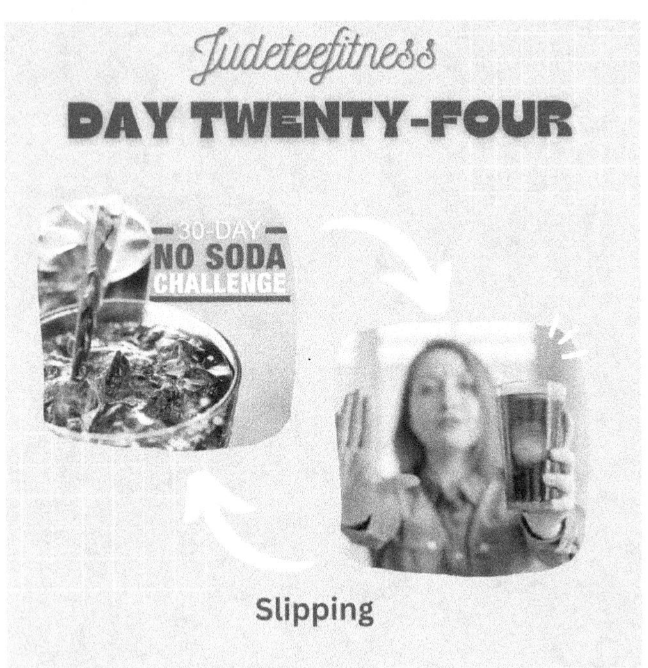

TWENTY-FOUR

Slipping

Don't beat yourself, but don't do it on purpose. Be intentional about it. However, while doing your challenge, if you slip, no biggie. Slipping means you're trying, which is what counts! You can get back on track for the rest of the day. I know some of you will love this part.

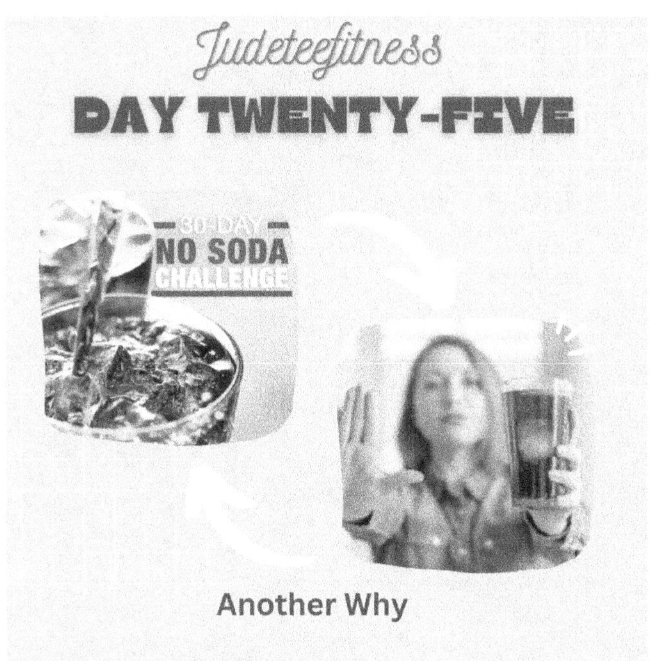

TWENTY-FIVE

Another Why

While researchers aren't sure of the precise reason, people
who drink pop are more likely to have osteoporosis.
A study published in Epidemiology indicates that drinking two
or more colas per day was associated with an increased risk of
chronic kidney disease.

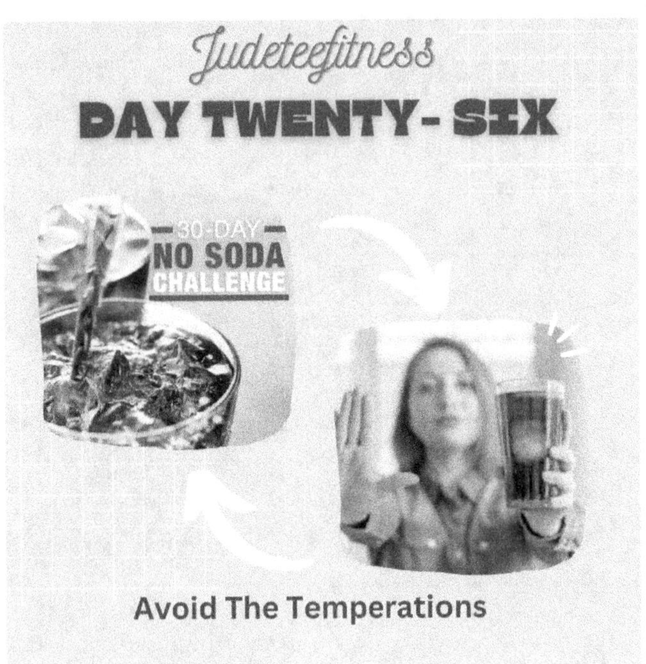

TWENTY-SIX

Avoid the Temptations

No doubt, you are already getting to the finish line, it is only normal to want to give a treat and say it doesn't matter. What you have started, you can finish. Just hold on and remember why you started at first.

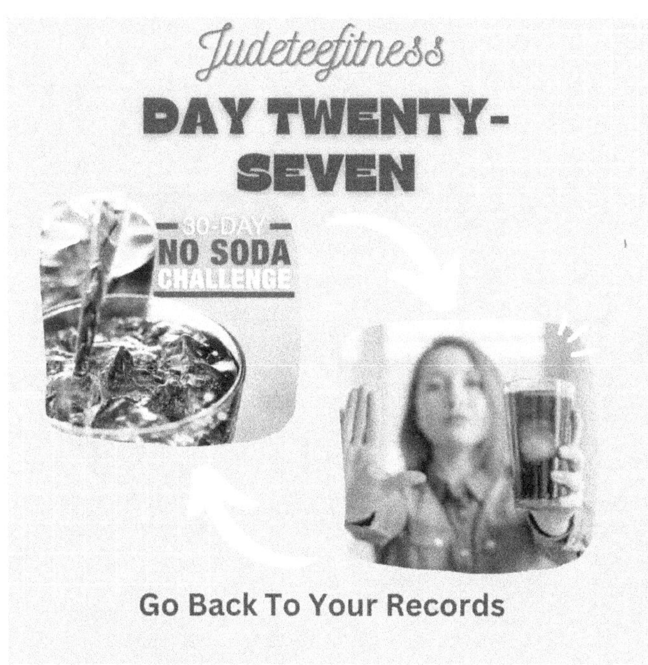

TWENTY-SEVEN

Go Back To Your Records.

Recall in day five we said something about keeping records because it helps you measure your progress. Go back to your record and see how far you've come. Identify those hurdles and hiccups you encountered and plan to work on them in your next challenge. Pat yourself in the back and know that you did it regardless.

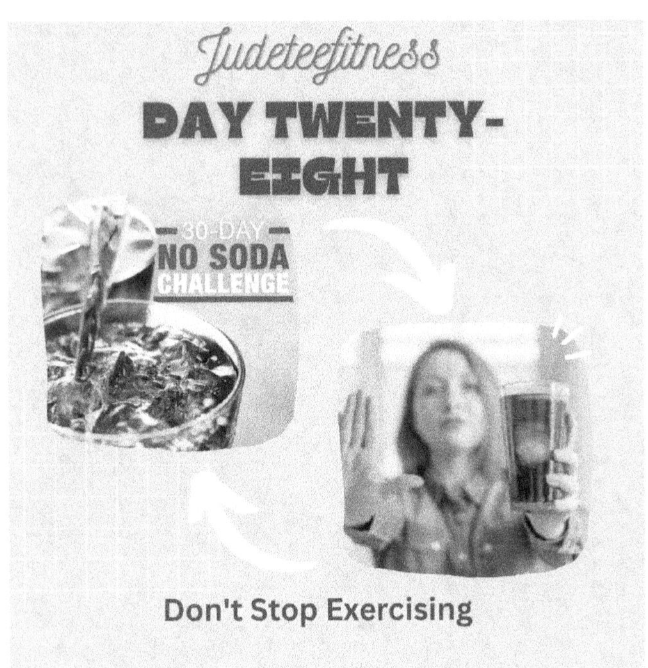

TWENTY-EIGHT

Don't Stop Exercising

Consistency is the key. Don't stop exercising, pick the days and times that will be suitable for you and engage consistently. The truth remains that fitness is a lifestyle and exercise not only helps you burn calories, but also makes you feel better.

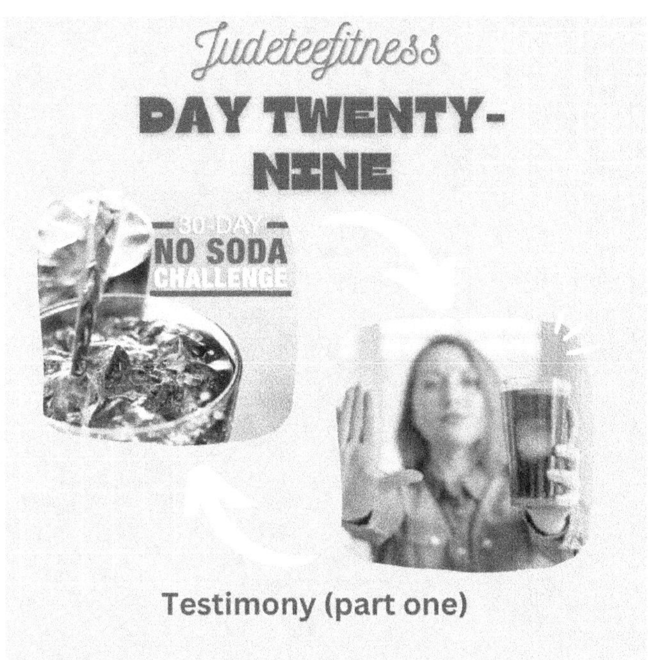

TWENTY-NINE

TESTIMONY (PART ONE)

I was also a soda addict, in fact, coca cola to be precise, I decided to challenge myself in 2020 to go without it for a year, I am proud to say I did it, in fact, my siblings will tempt me with it so much, they were shocked I refused to take it. 1 month should be a walk in the park for me, if I can set my mind to staying off soda for 1 year then I think I can do anything I set my mind to do. - **JESSICA**

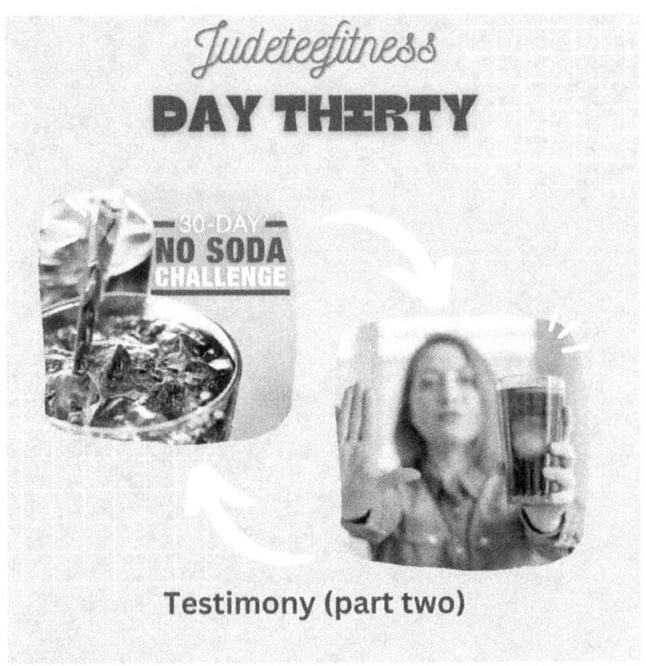

Testimony (part two)

THIRTY

TESTIMONY (PART TWO)

I was tempted today, it was a hectic day. I traveled to Bomadi then to ogbe-Ijoh back to Sapele. on our way back we went to get something to eat, I told my colleague what I need right now is a cold bottle of Pepsi, she said yes and ordered one and asked how far, I said "No, I'm on 30 days No soda challenge" and she said be fooling yourself, who will know if you take or not. Well, I said I didn't join the challenge for the group but for myself. I requested a bottle of water instead - **GWEKE**

CONCLUSION

In conclusion, you have to gain control over your body. Being motivated to smash your fitness challenge is a long-term goal as such you should first deal with the mind. Remember to give yourself flexibility and celebrate the little successes along your journey. Please, don't be afraid to ask for help when needed.

With the proper tools and support from your partner or group, you can stay motivated to reach your goals. Wish you success.

30 MINDSETS

THAT WILL MAKE YOU SMASH A NO-SODA/FITNESS CHALLENGE WITH EASE

Most people certainly wonder how fitness models and celebrities achieve so much in their fitness lives, the tips and tricks. Do you know? 8 out of 10 successful people, on average, start from the mindset they have. The success mindset is the initial capital to get a successful life. Not only successful but also a happier person. However, to smash your no-soda/fitness challenge, I have written everything in this book.

ABOUT THE AUTHOR

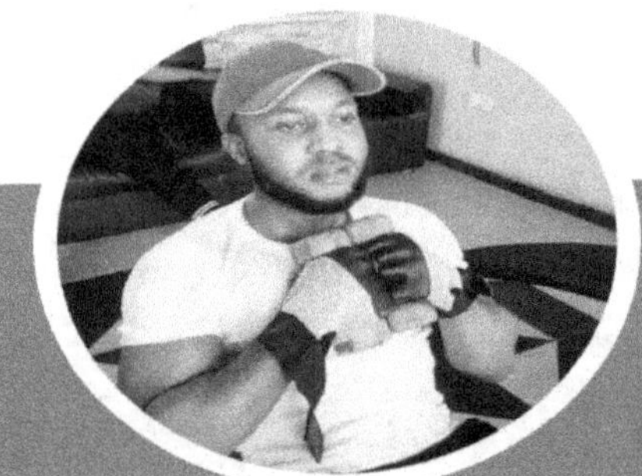

Jude Aghwaremre

Jude is a graduate of mathematics and statistics from the University of Calabar. So far, he has focused on researching self-development and is passionate about helping people achieve their fitness goals. He is a certified virtual assistant, health and fitness creator, and massage detox specialist. From his research experience and love for fitness, he has organized different programs and finally launched this book to help people maximize their potential.